I0436208

Copyright © 2014 by Sean Jackson

All rights reserved. No part of this book may
be reproduced or transmitted in any form or
by any means, electronic or mechanical,
including photocopying, recording, or by any
information storage and retrieval system
without the written permission of the author,
except where permitted by law.

Printed in the United States of America

First Edition, 2014

ISBN 978-1494904609

Dedicated to my niece Emersyn

Spud was a potato from a town much like yours.

He lived on a street
in a house with blue doors

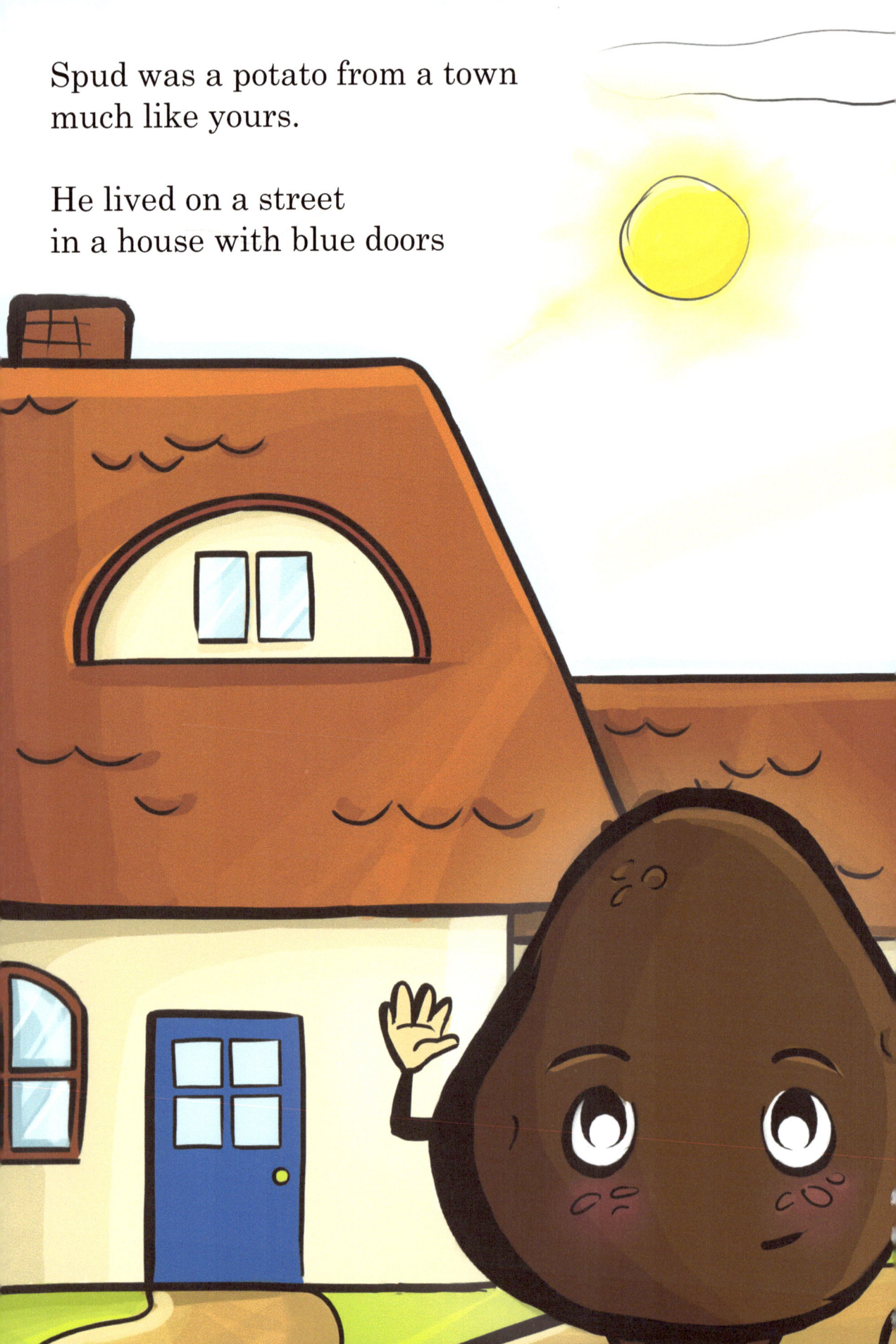

Spud had a family,
a sister and brother.

A fry was his dad and a
sweet potato pie was his mother.

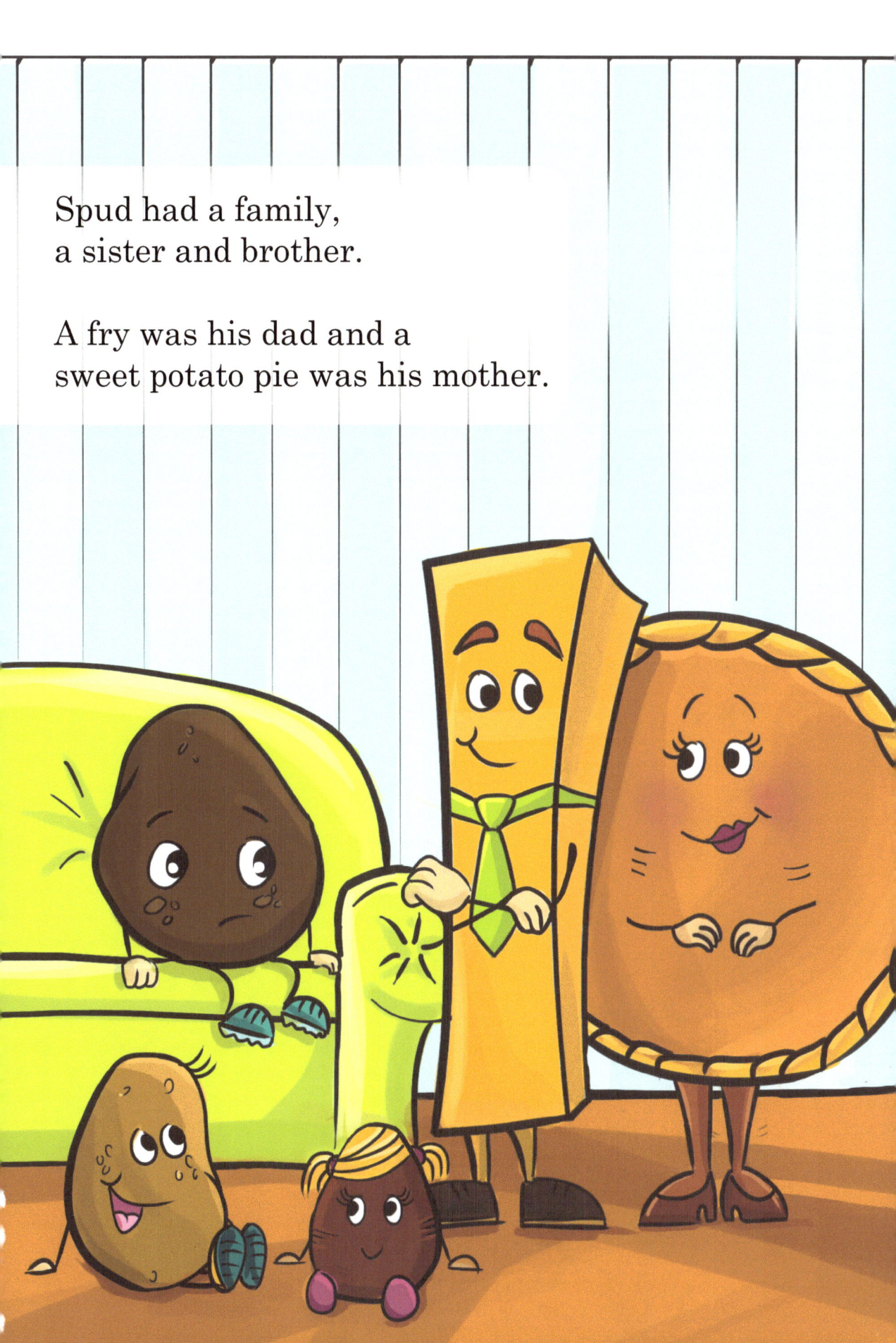

But Spud had a problem.
He was a bit of a grouch.

His only interest in life
was to sit on his couch.

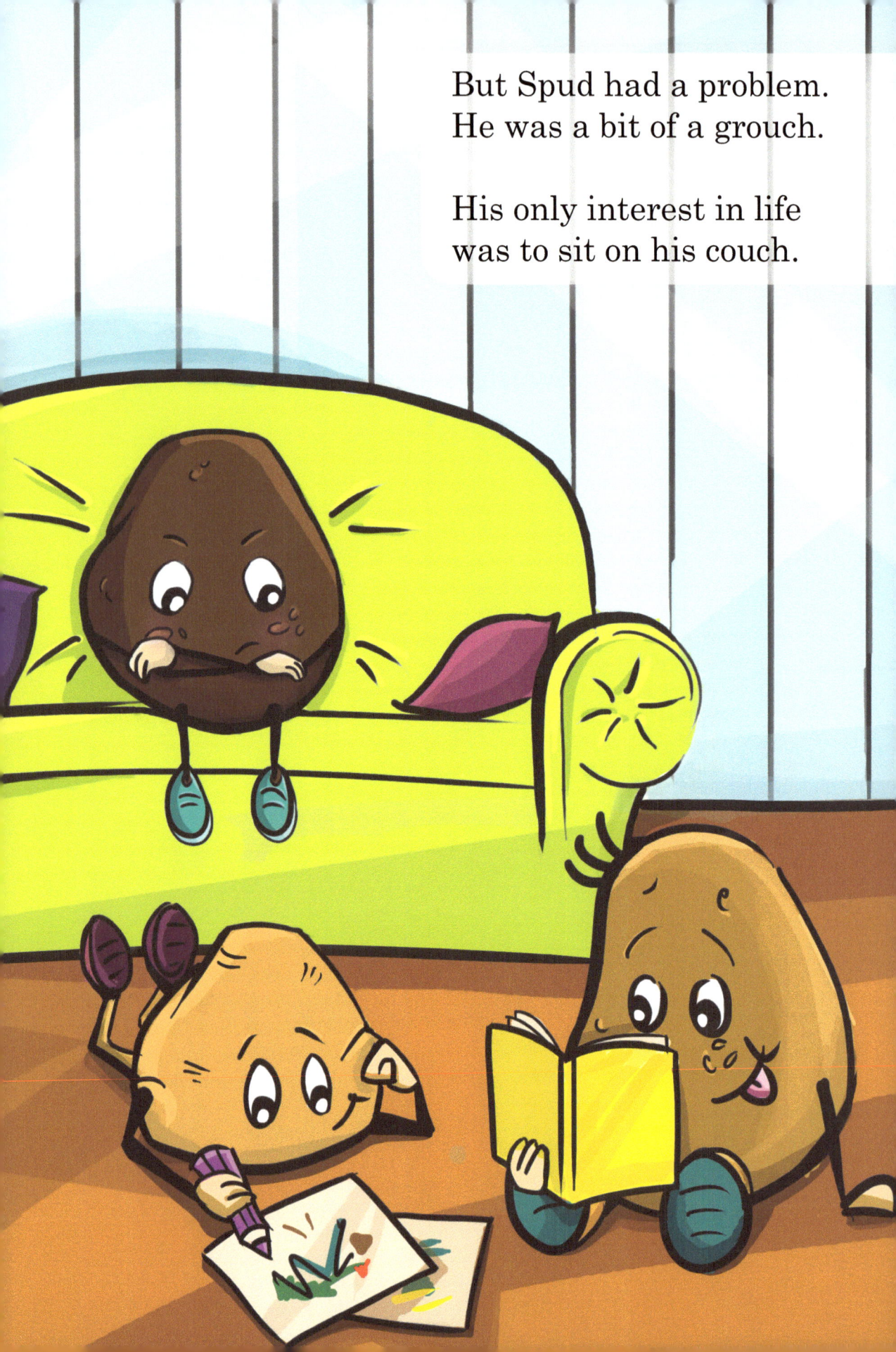

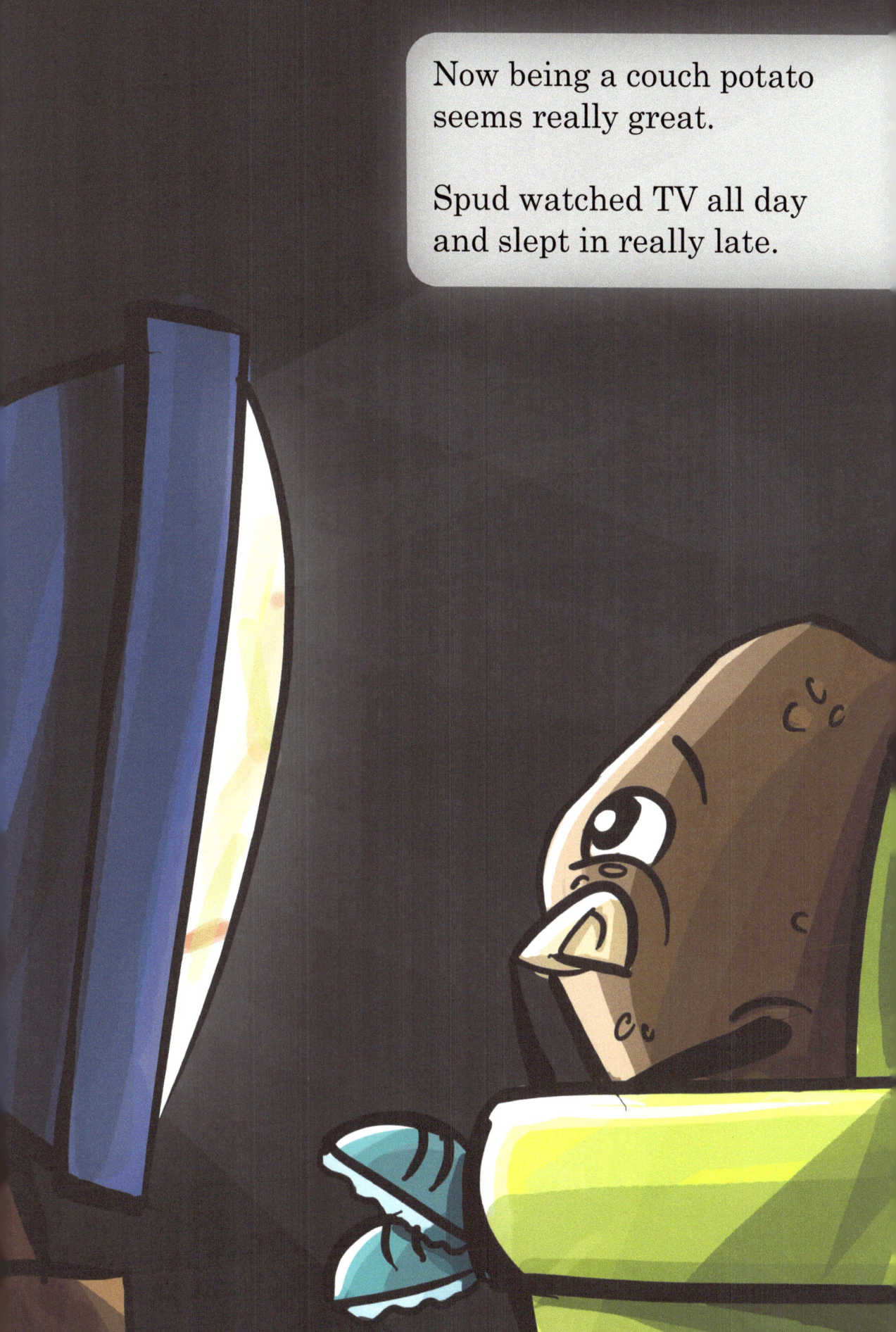

Now being a couch potato seems really great.

Spud watched TV all day and slept in really late.

Spud never jumped rope
or spent time with his friends.

He never read books
or painted pictures of hens.

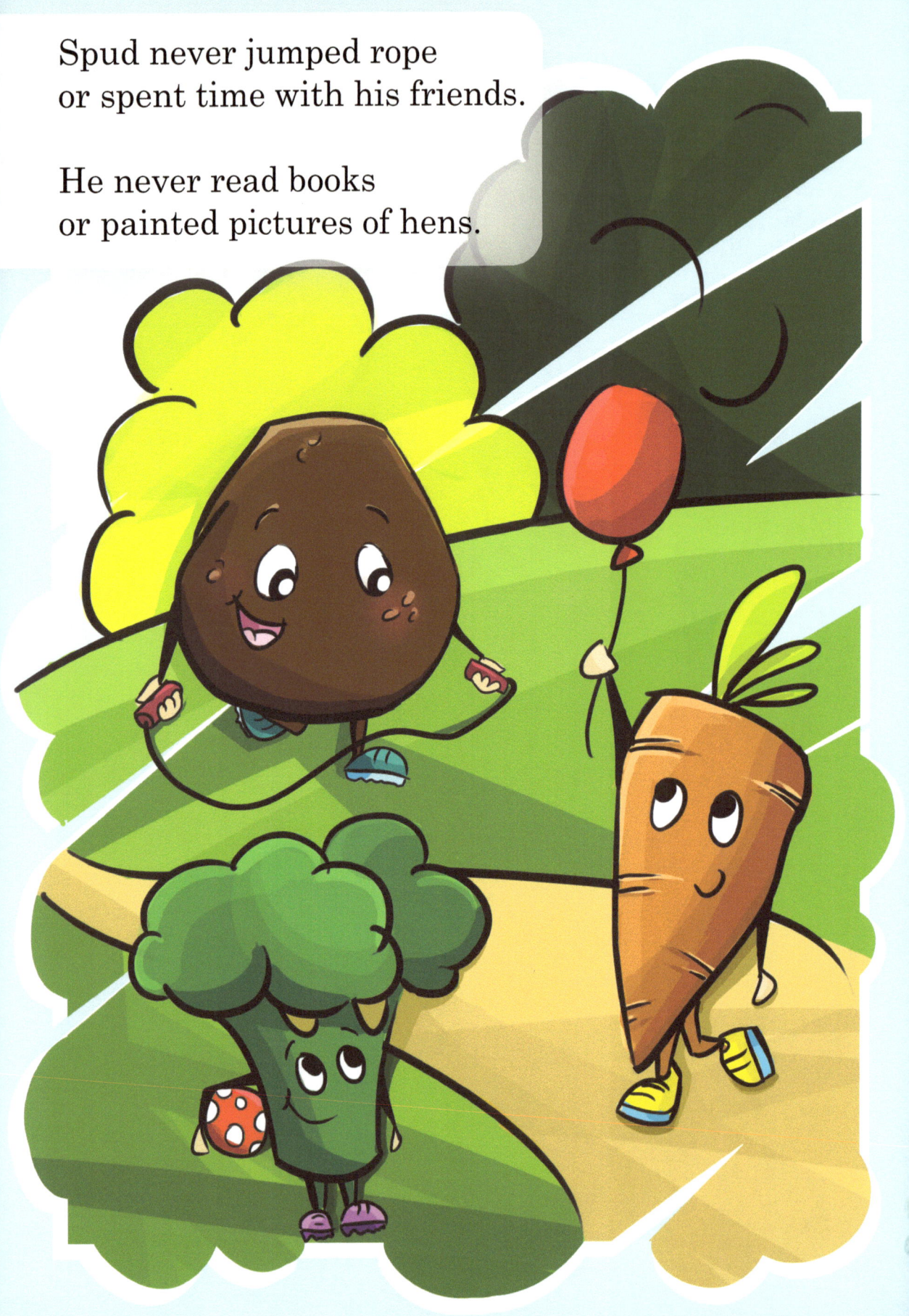

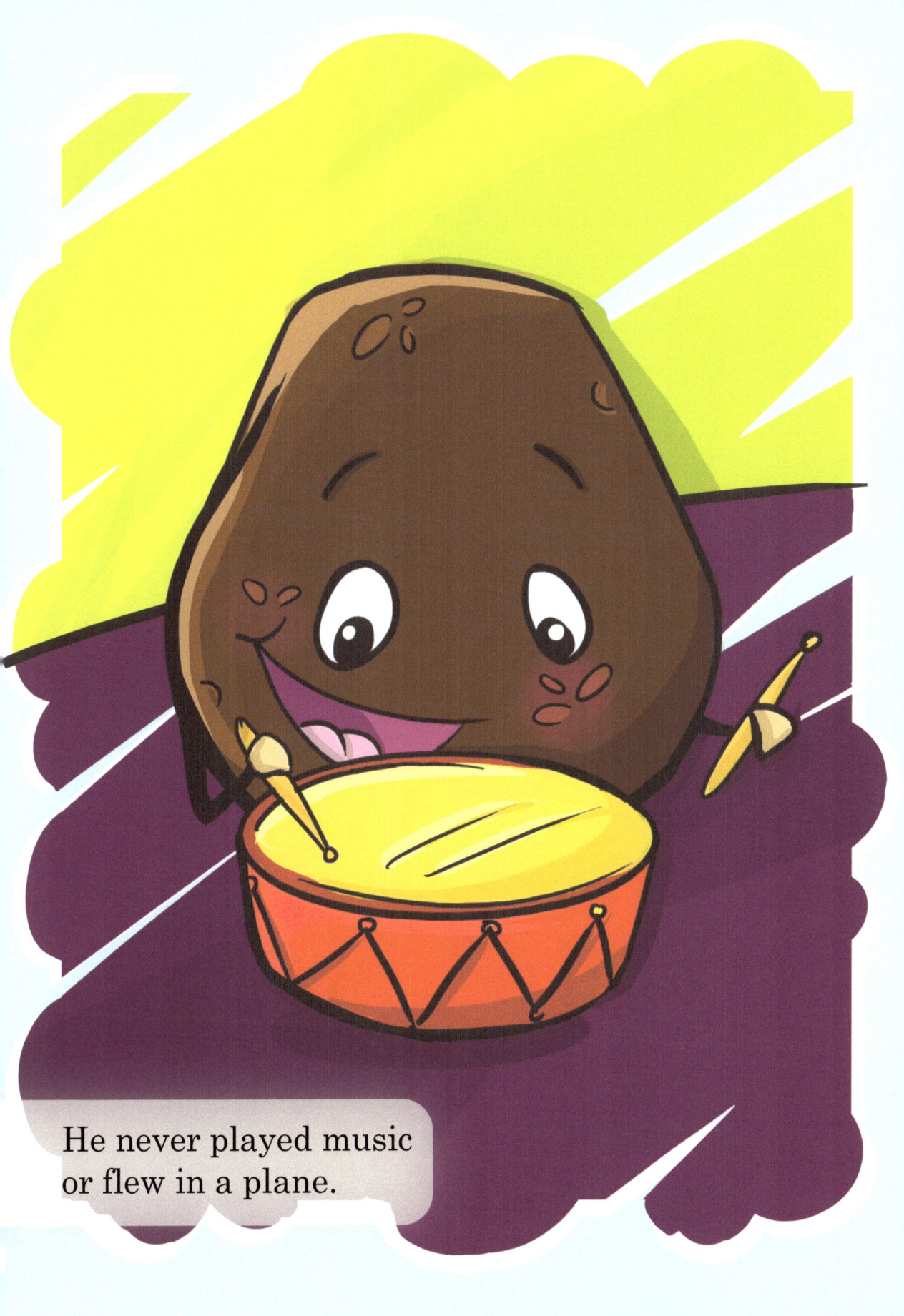

He never played music
or flew in a plane.

He never played baseball or rode on a train.

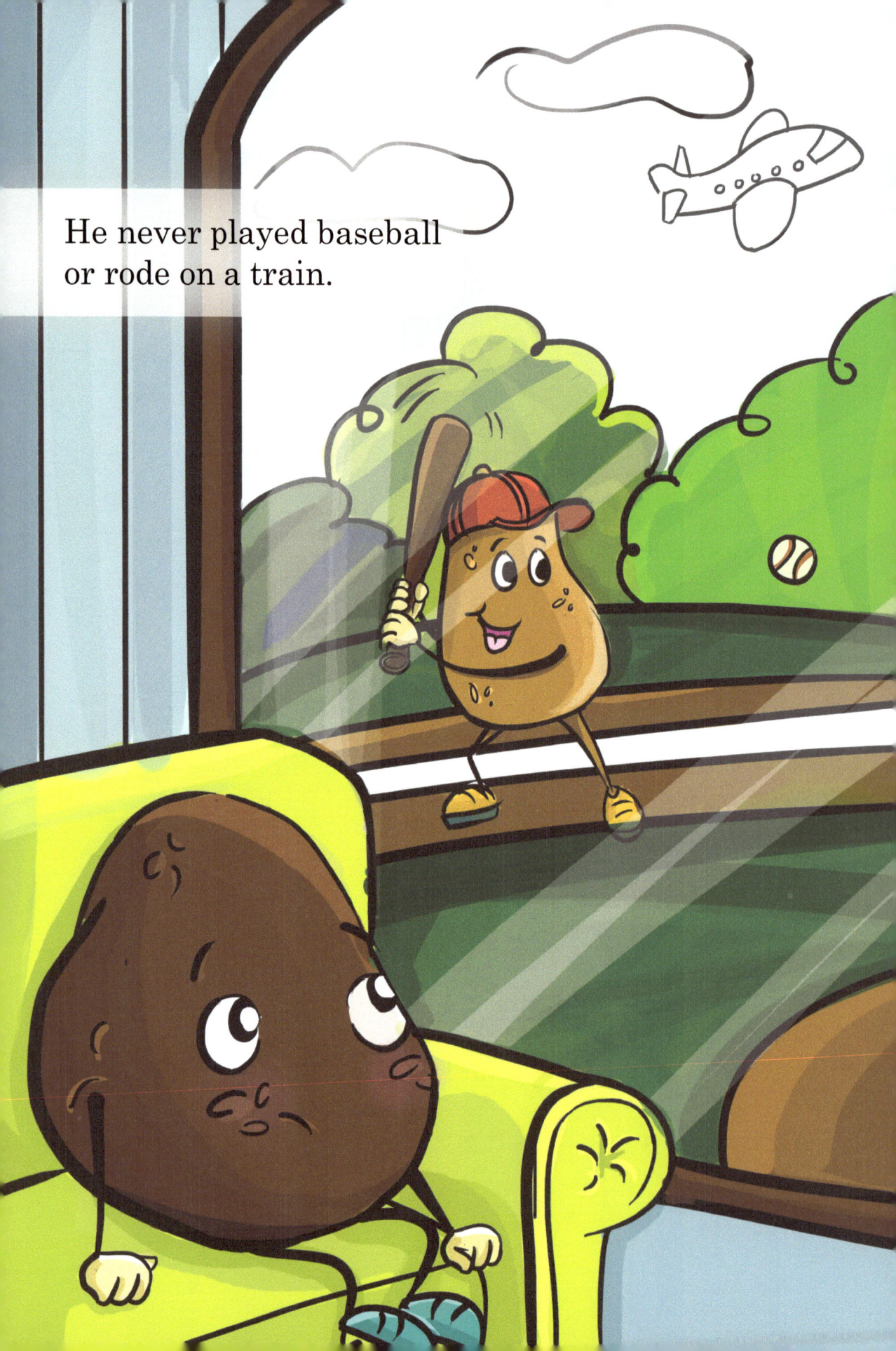

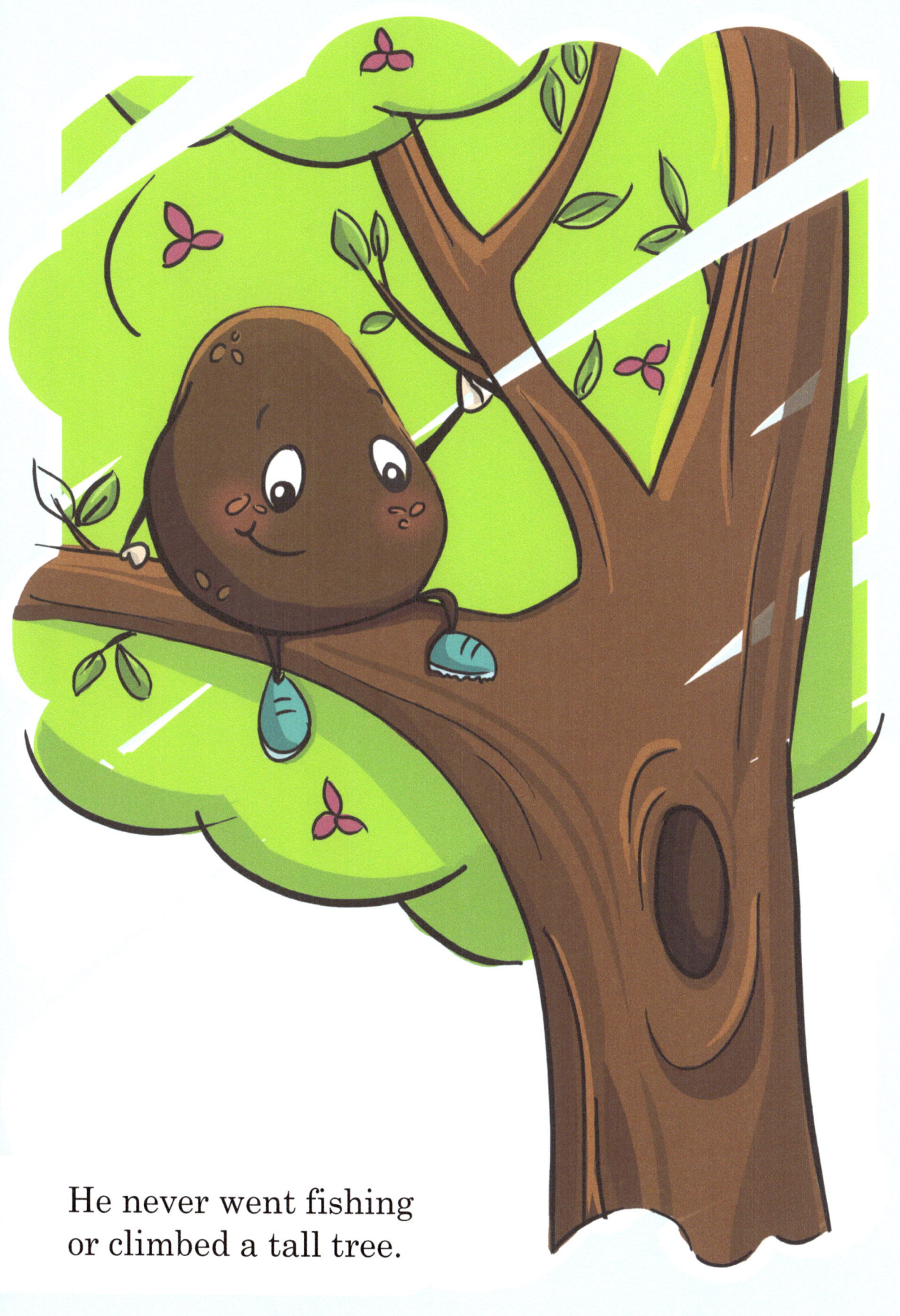

He never went fishing
or climbed a tall tree.

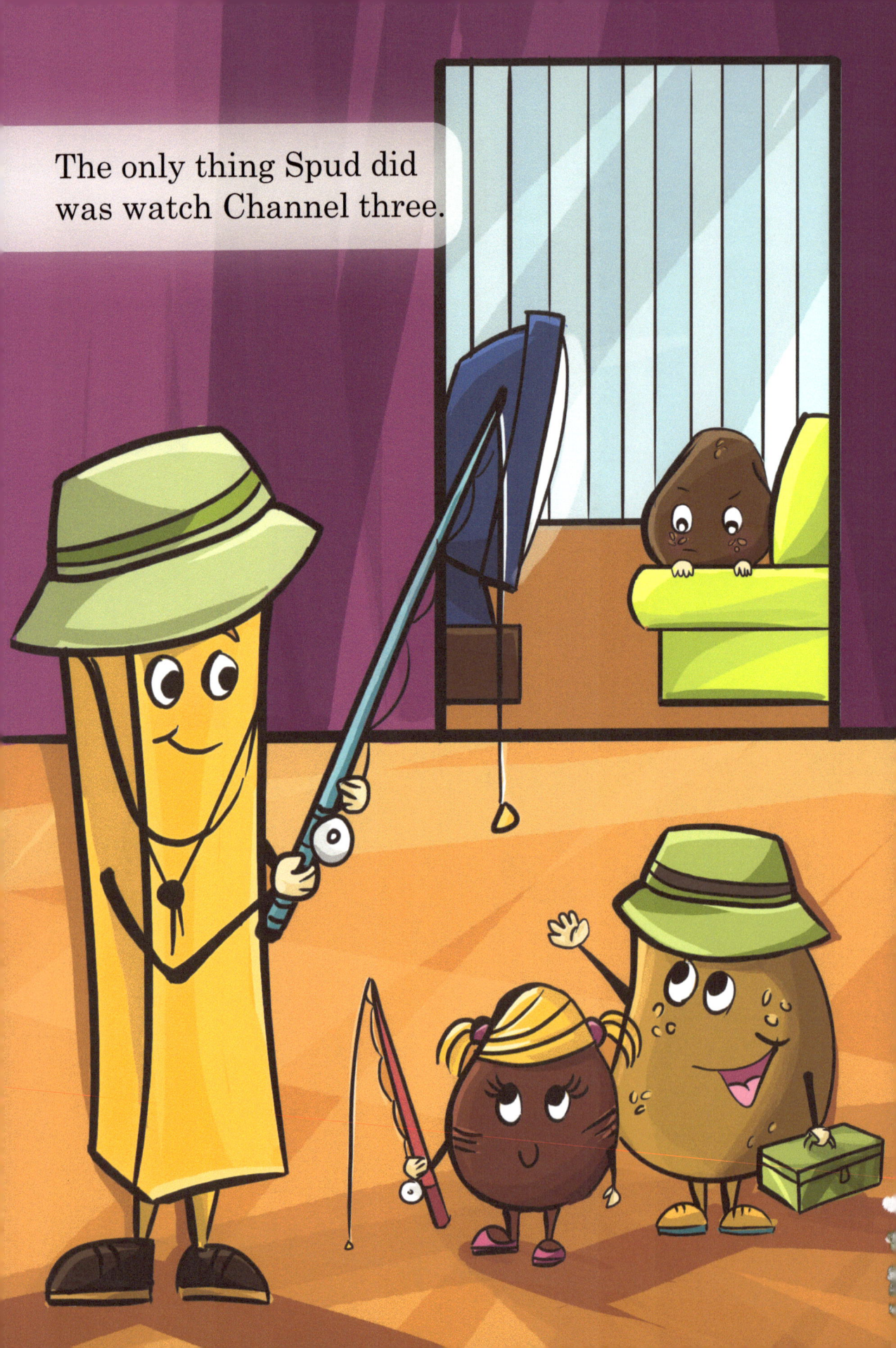

The only thing Spud did was watch Channel three.

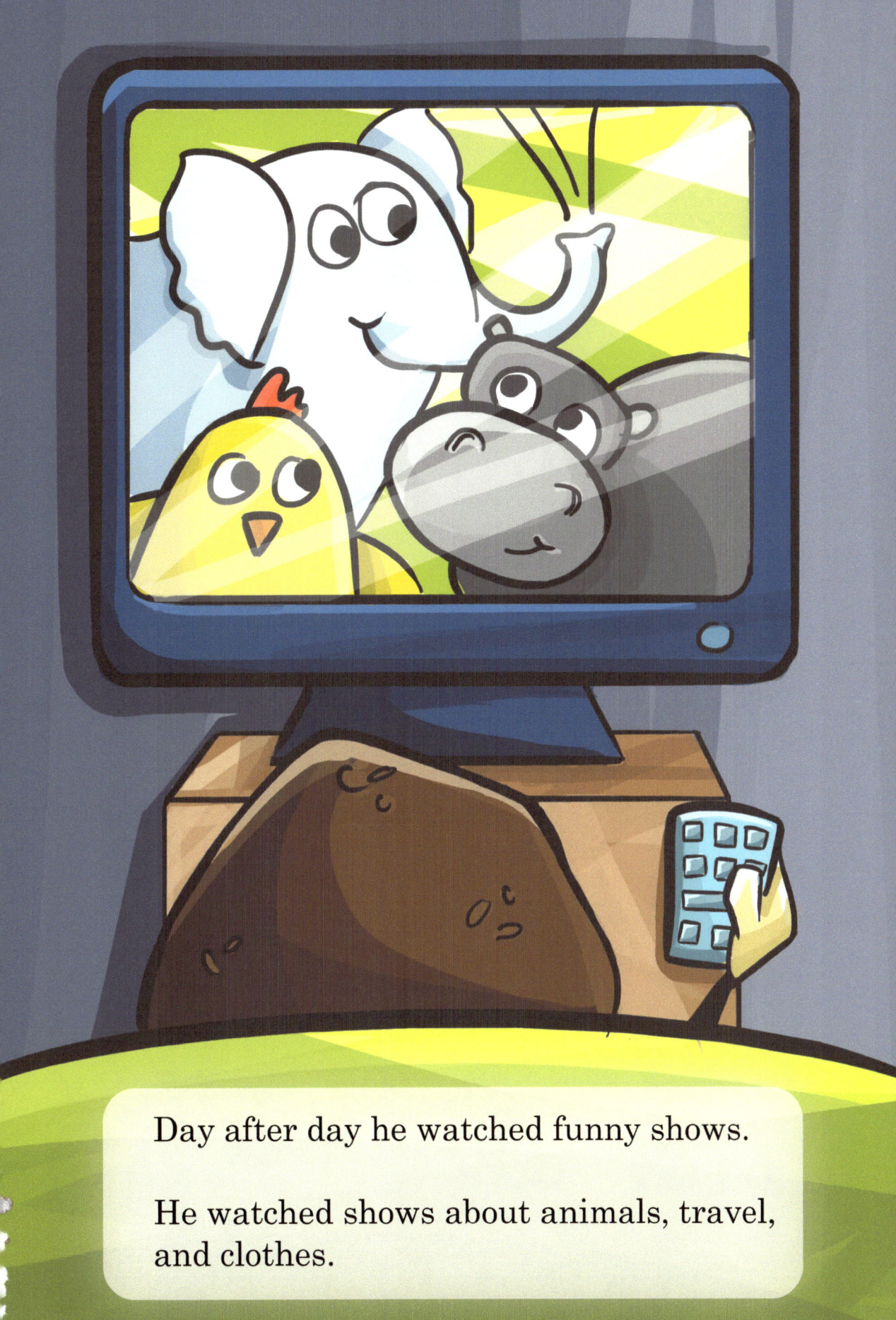

Day after day he watched funny shows.

He watched shows about animals, travel, and clothes.

He watched cartoons about cowboys and rockets in space.

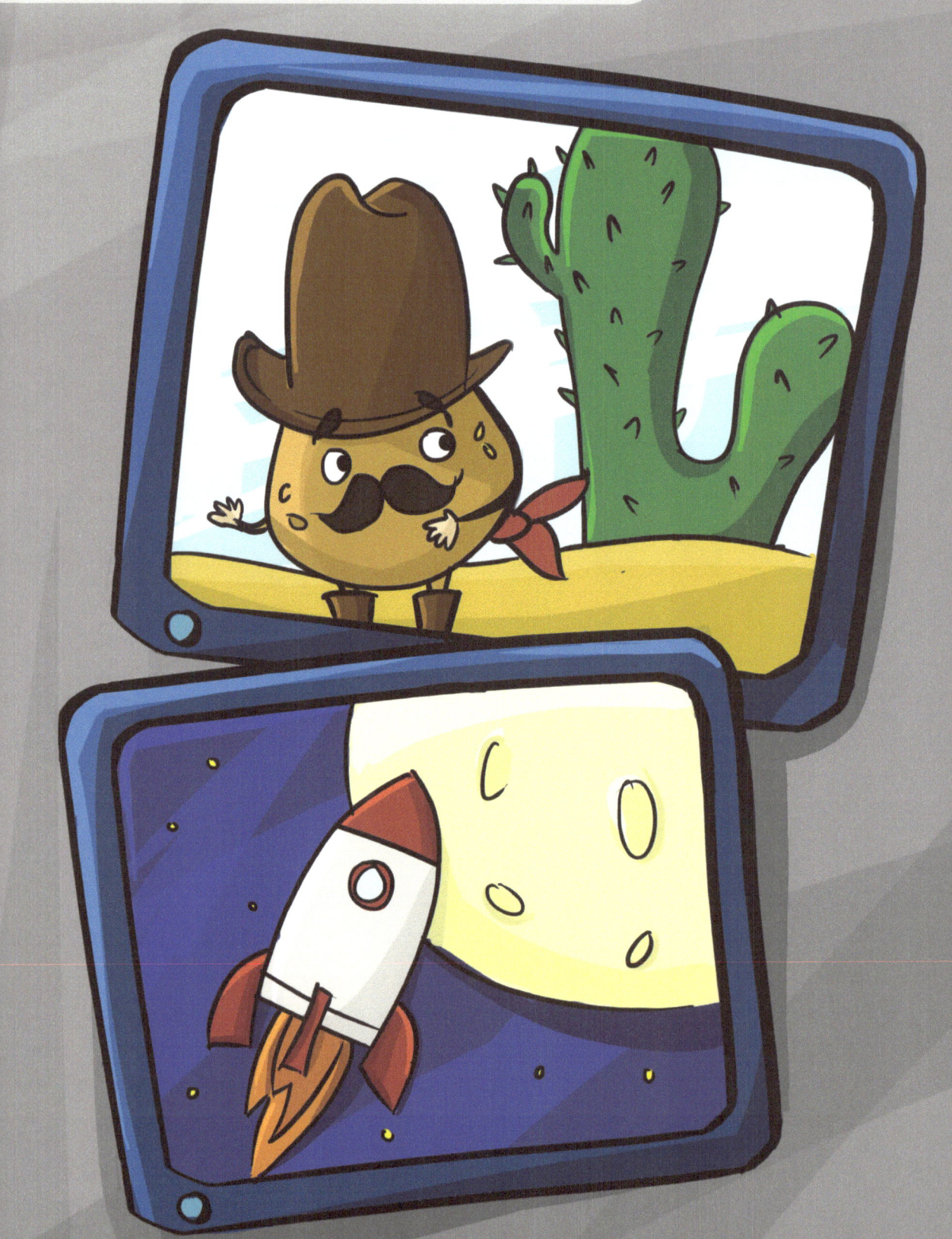

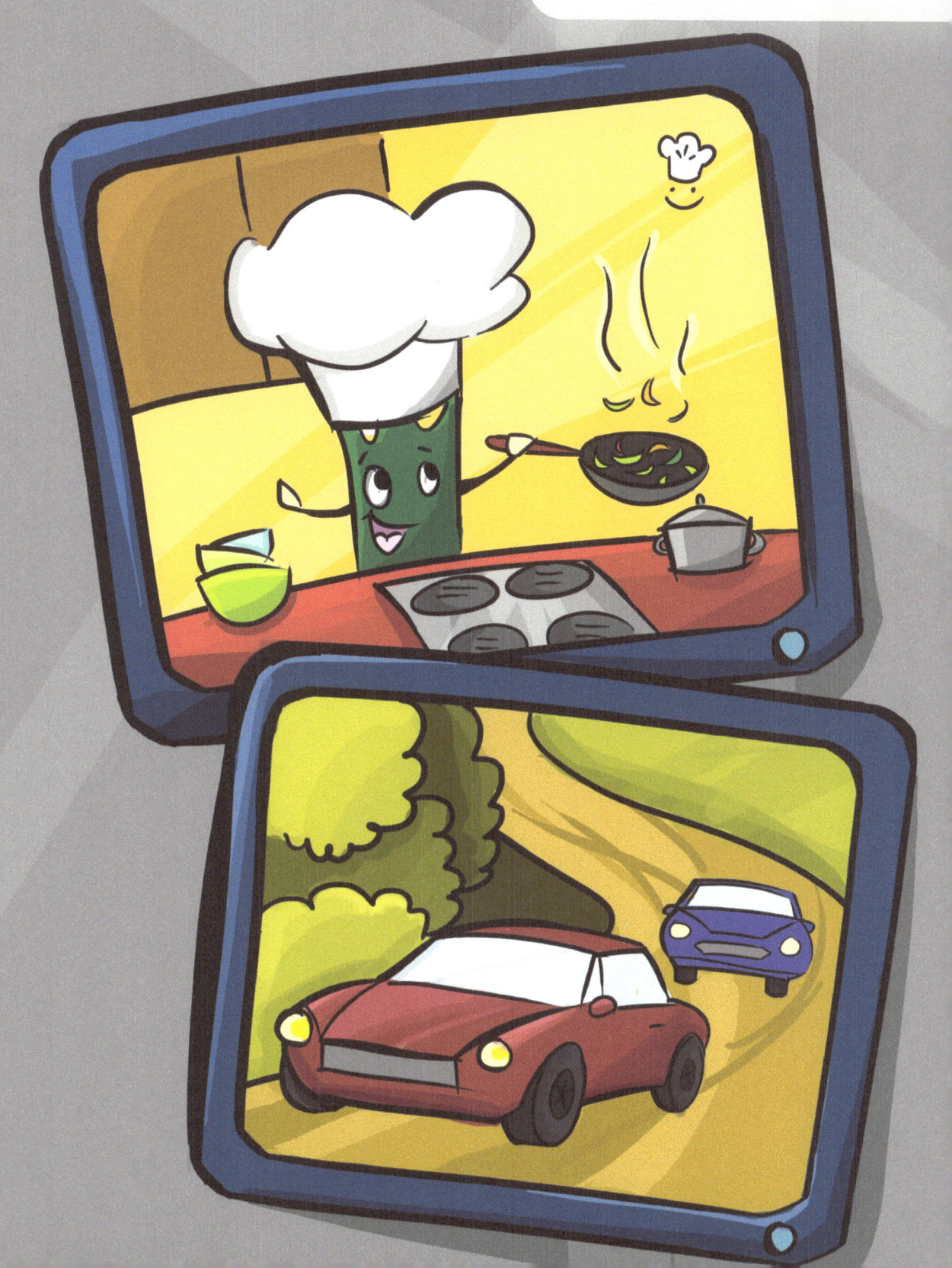

Shows about cooking and cars in a chase.

Then something happened one terrible day.

The TV went black and Spuds shows went away.

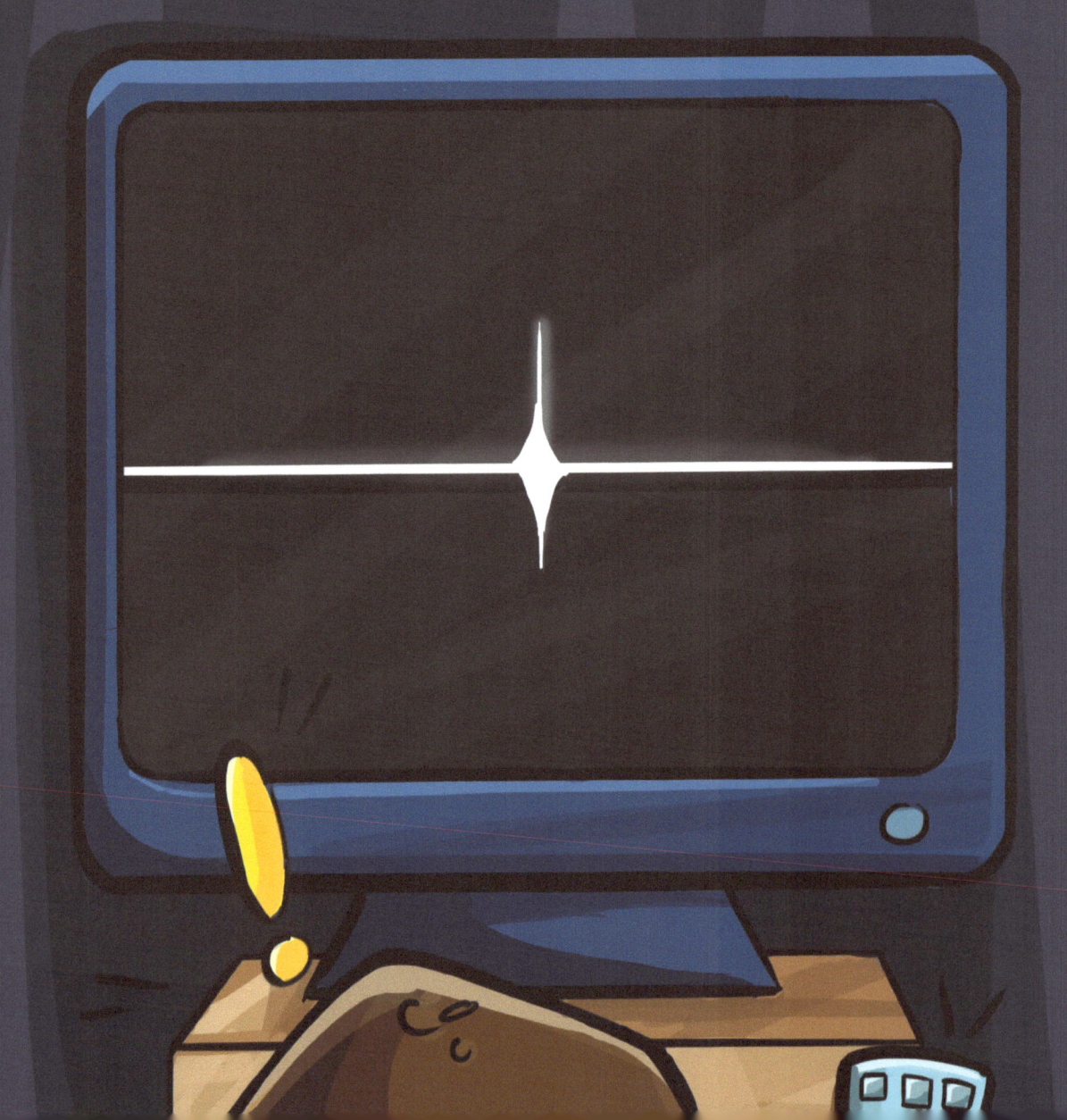

He cried and he howled
"How can this be?!"

"What will I do
without my TV?"

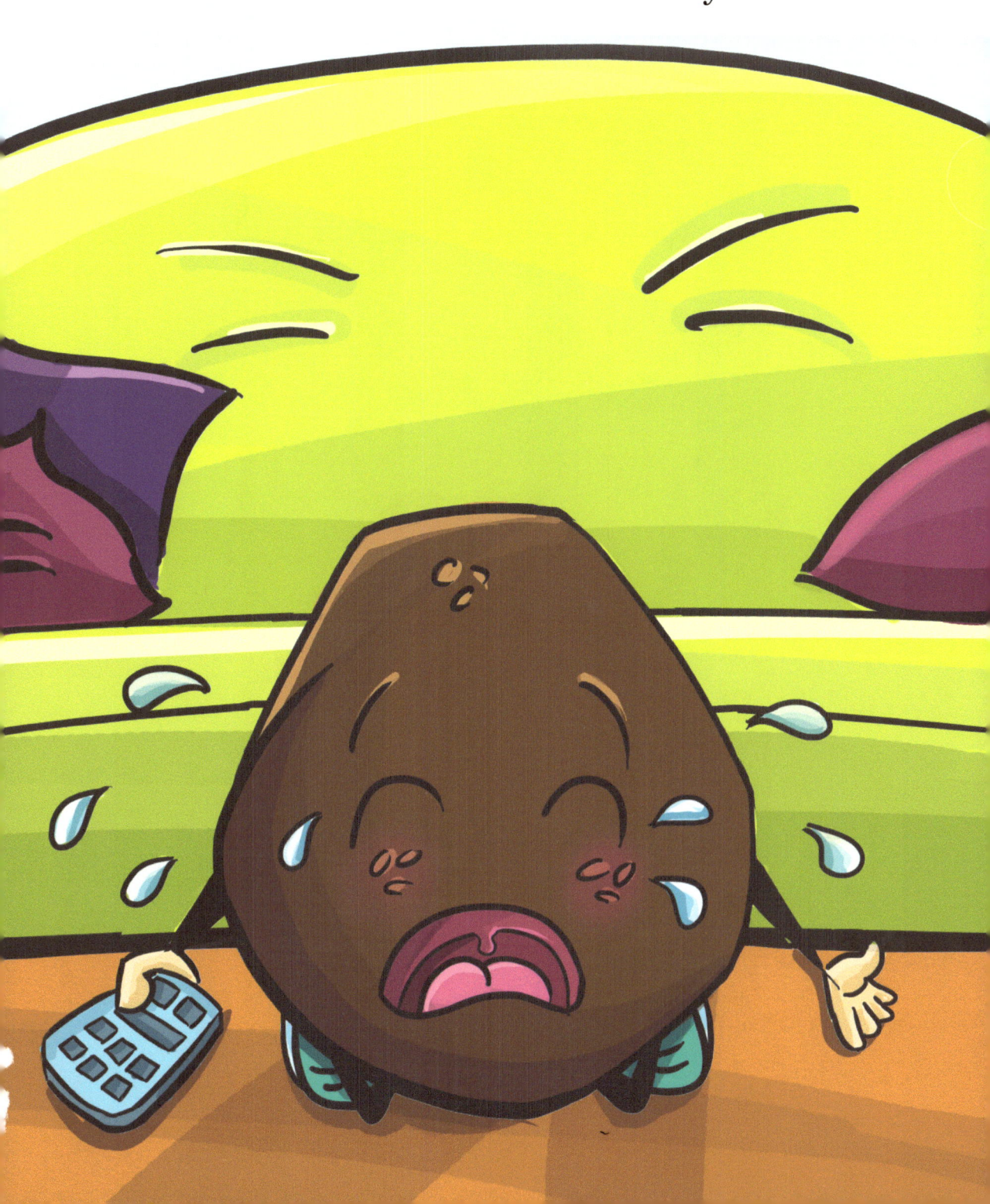

Spud had no choice
but to get on his feet.

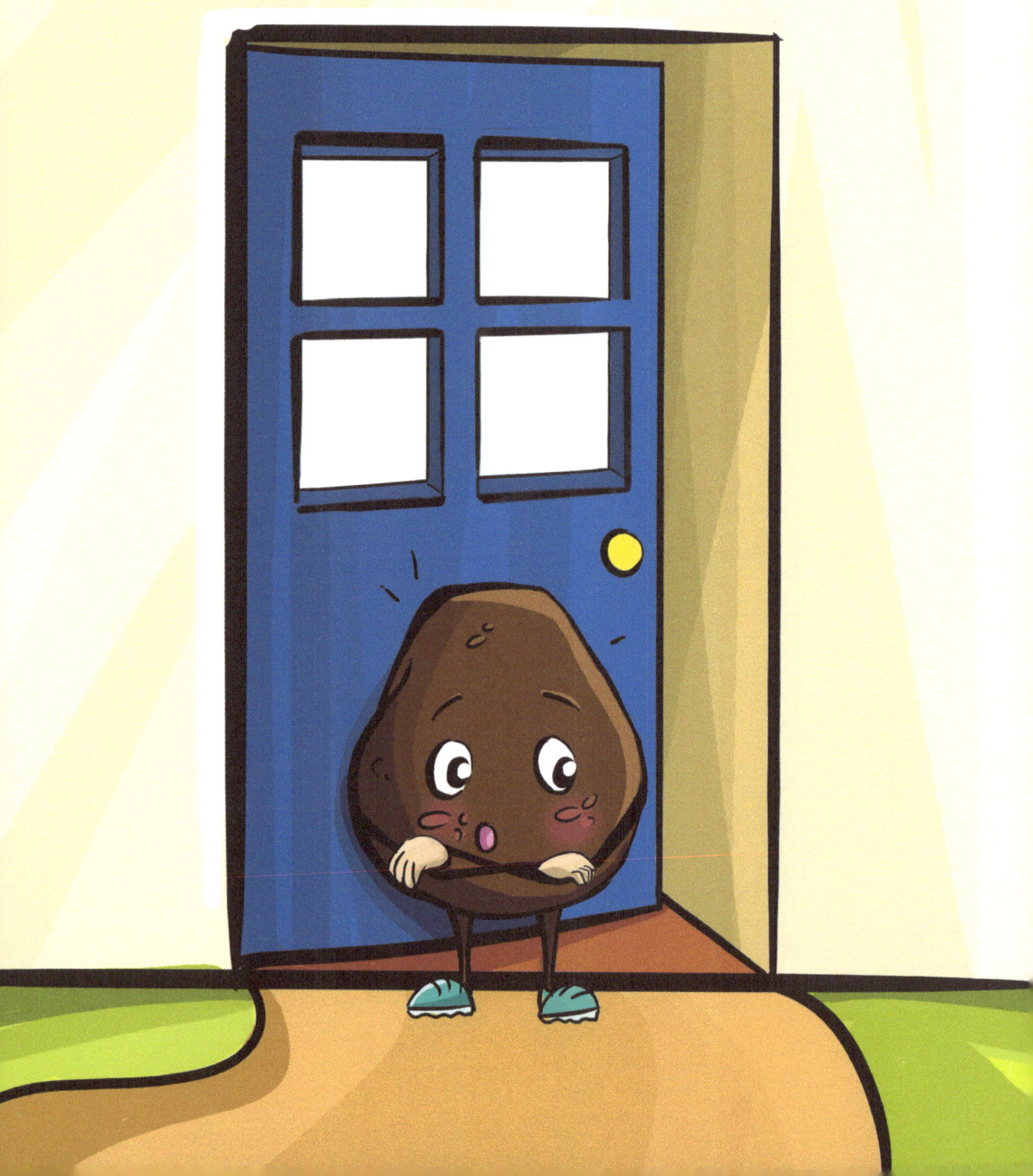

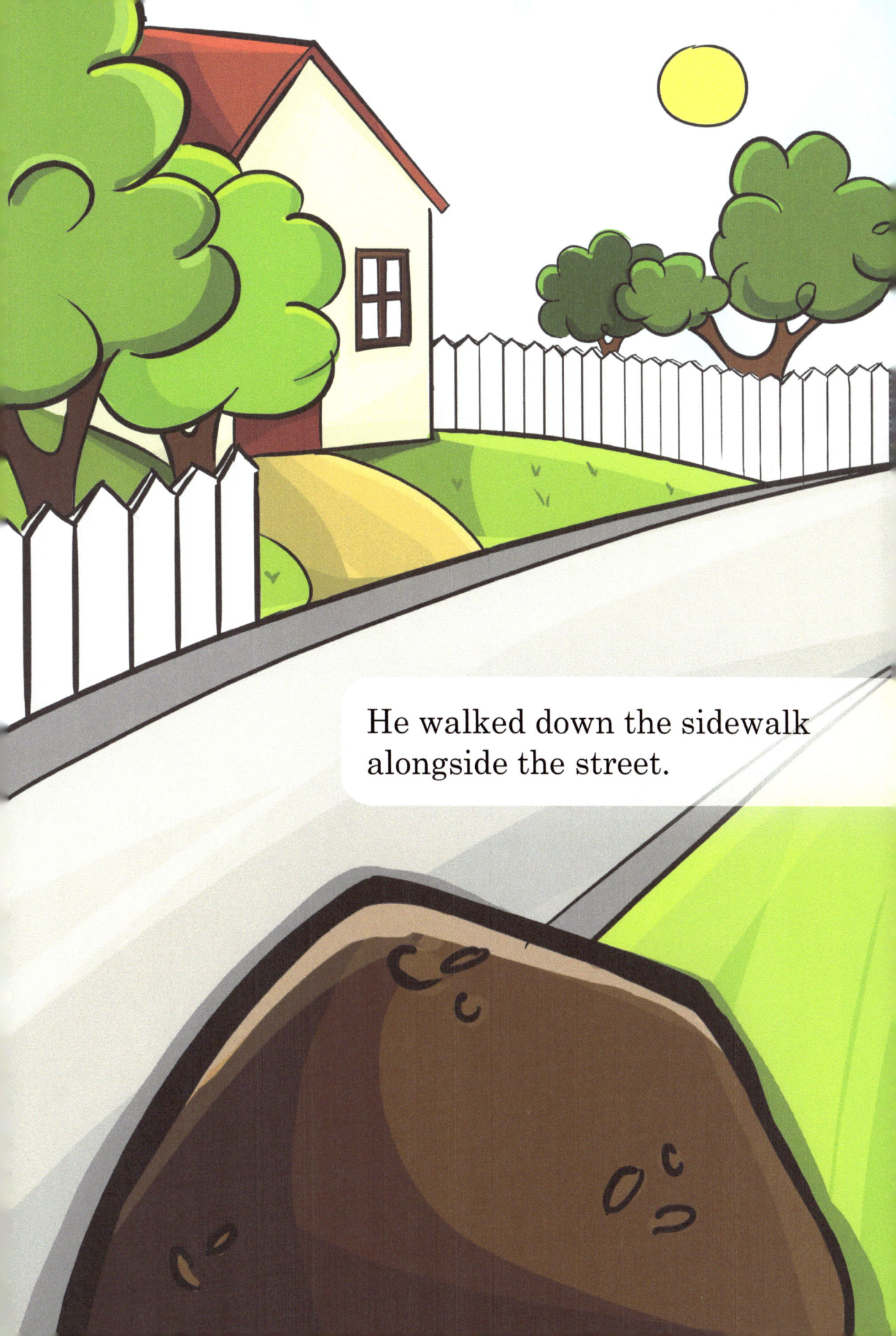

He walked down the sidewalk alongside the street.

Outside some young taters were playing baseball.

"Come play with us Spud!" he heard them all call.

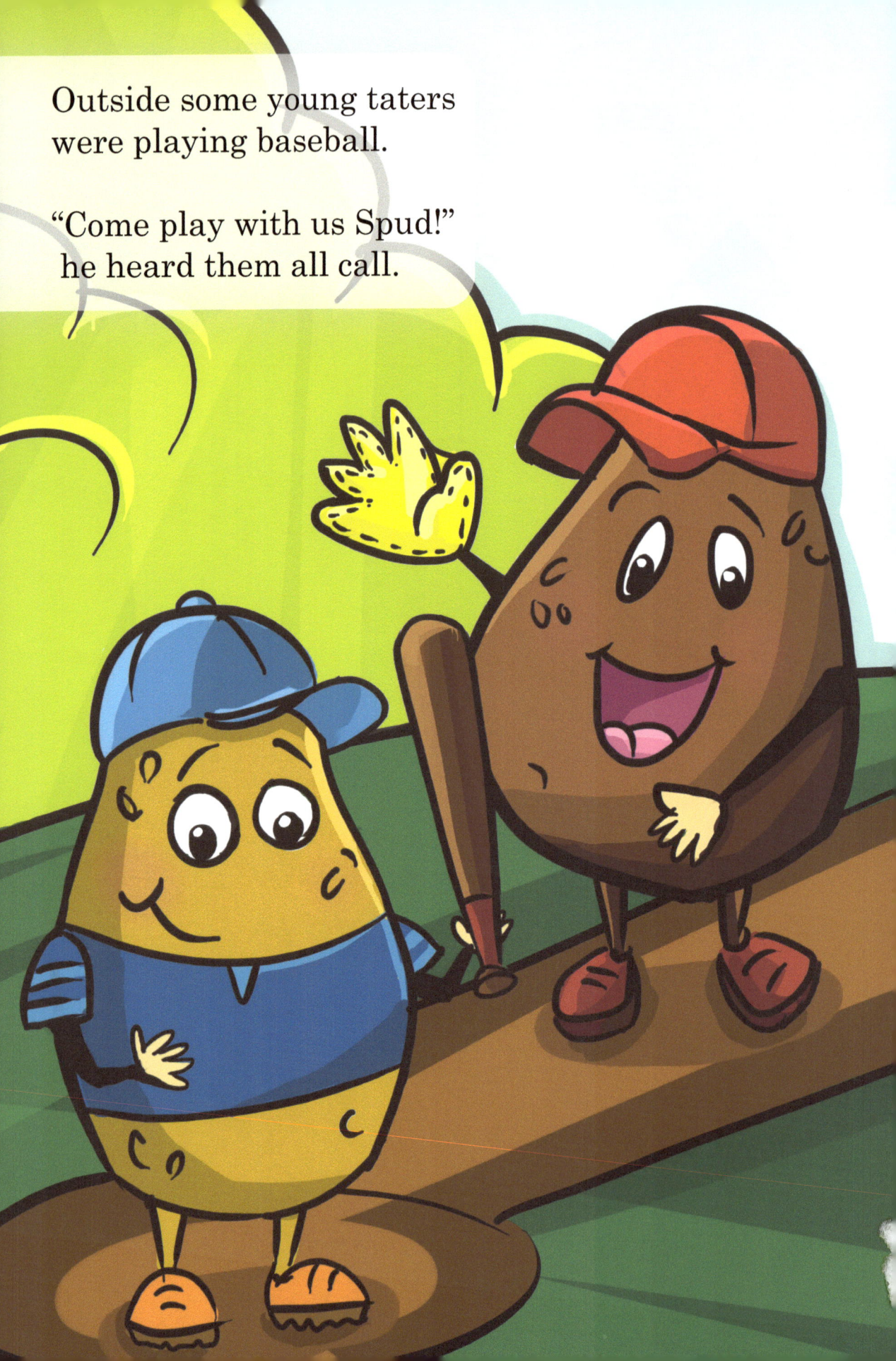

Spud didn't want to.
Not one little bit.

Playing was tiresome.
He'd much rather sit.

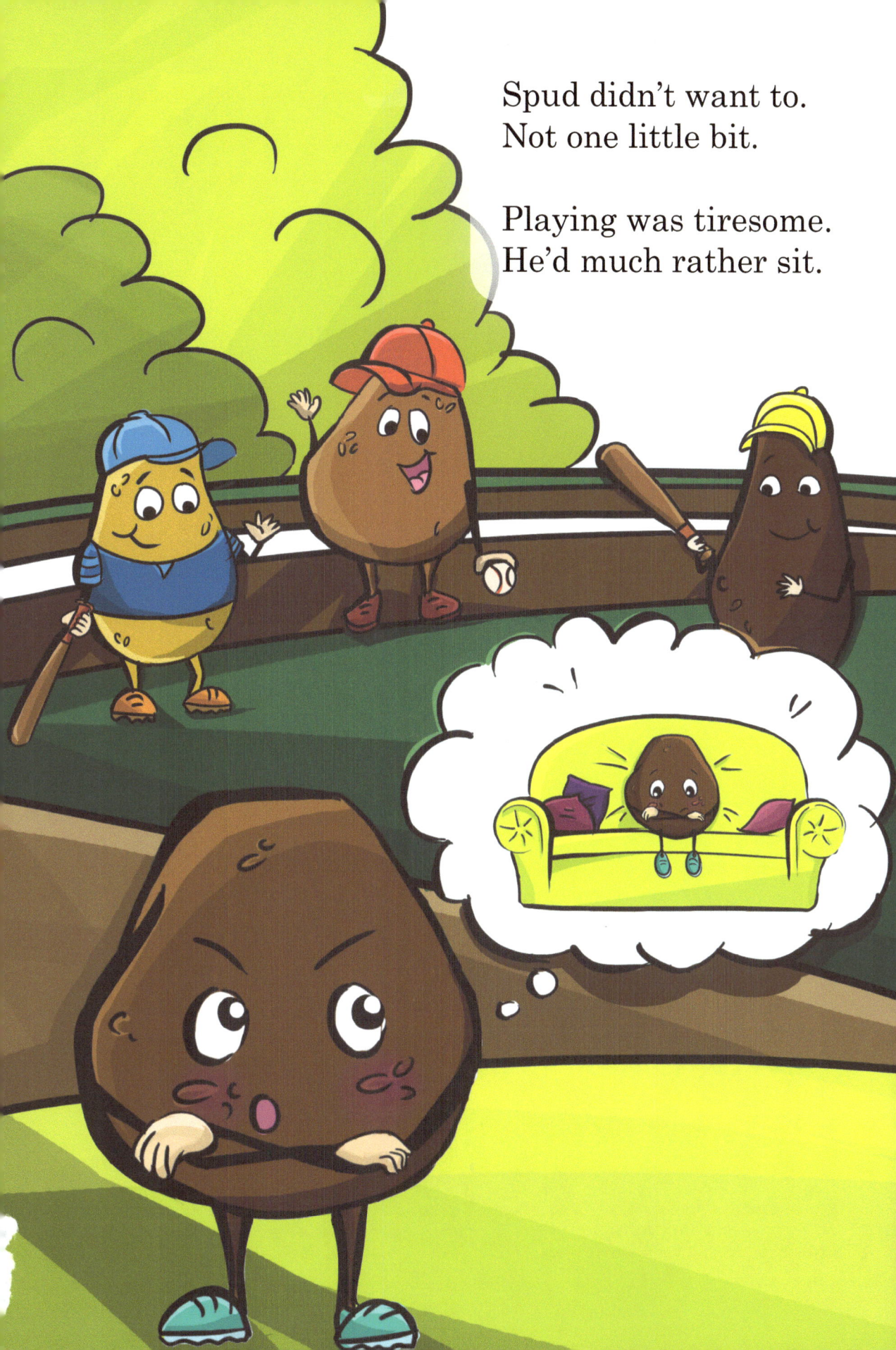

"I've never played baseball."
Spud said with a sigh.

"It's OK, we can teach you.
Come give it a try!"

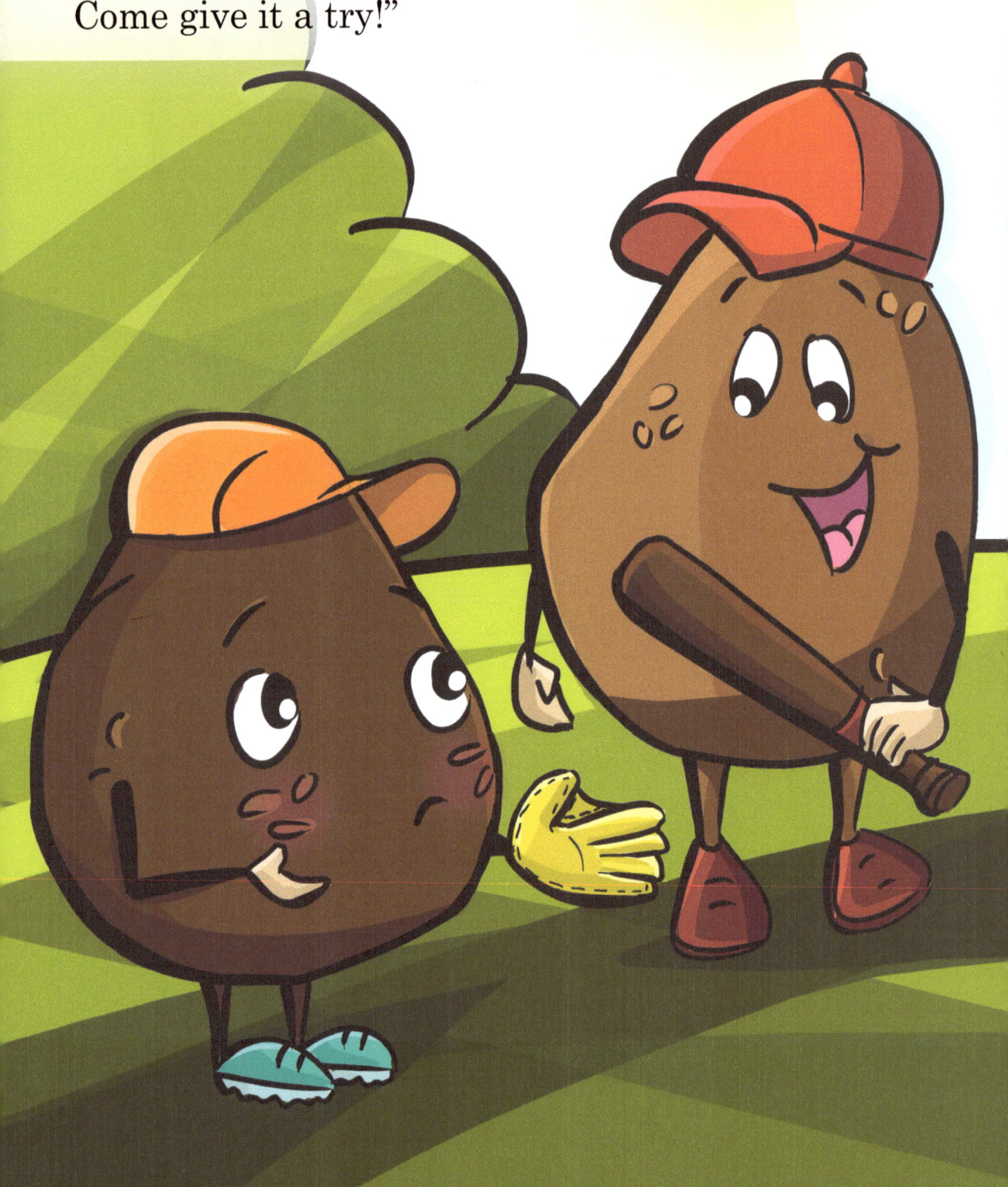

So they taught him to throw
and gave him a mitt.

Then he picked up a bat
and they taught him to hit.

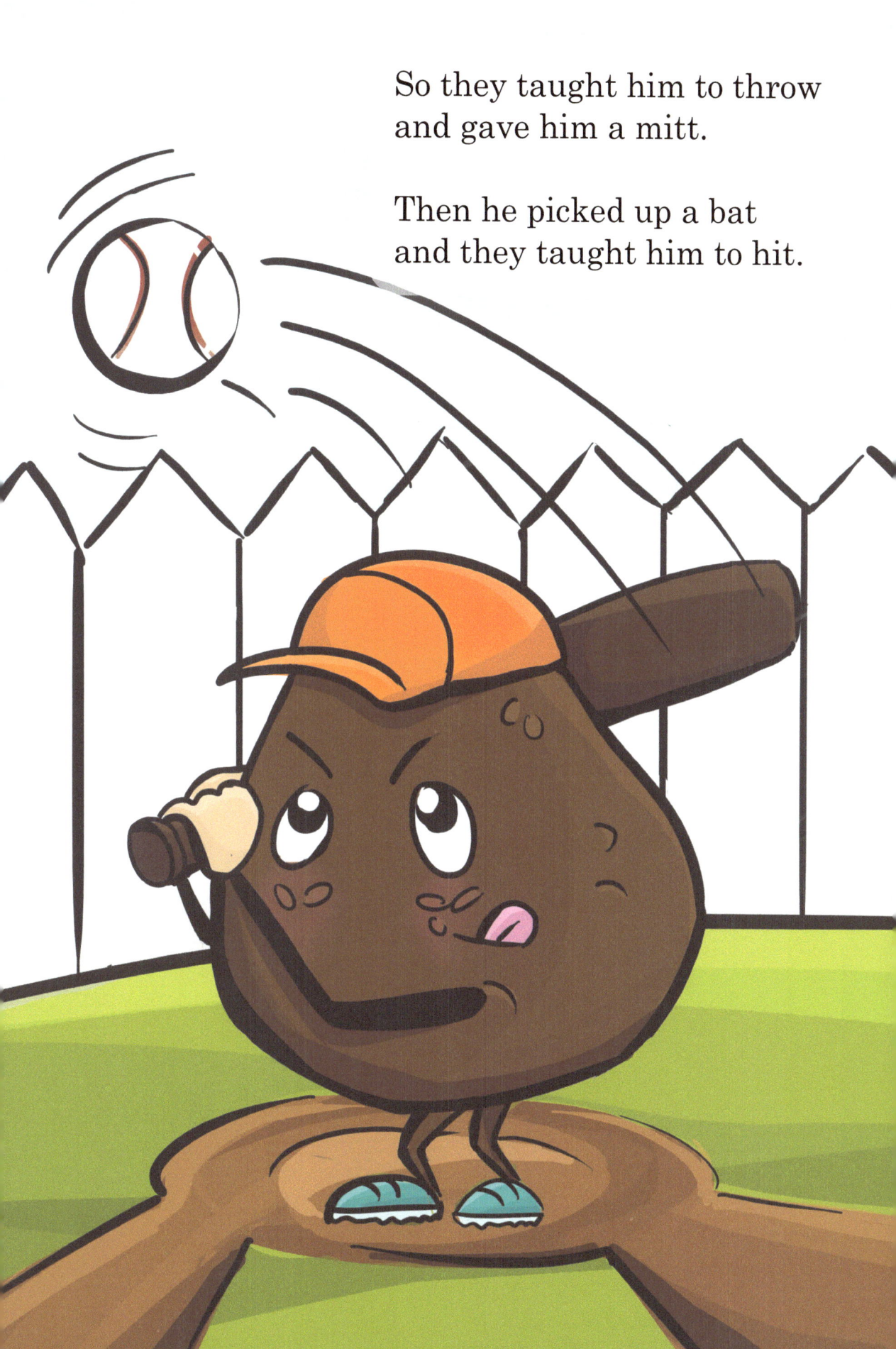

Spud was amazed
by the fun that he had.

"This playing outside
stuff isn't so bad."

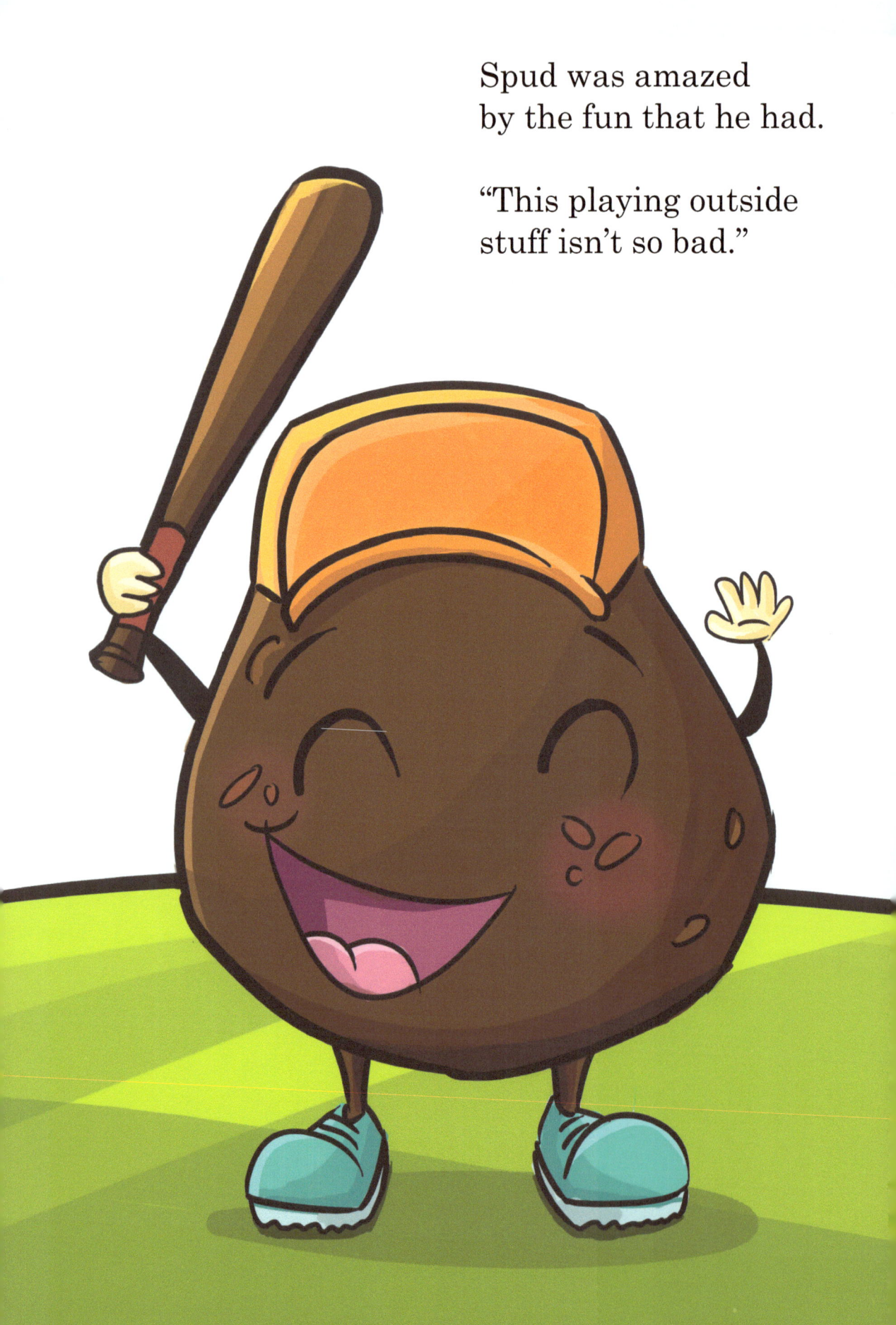

"I've been wasting my time watching so much TV."

He said with a smile as his heart filled with glee.

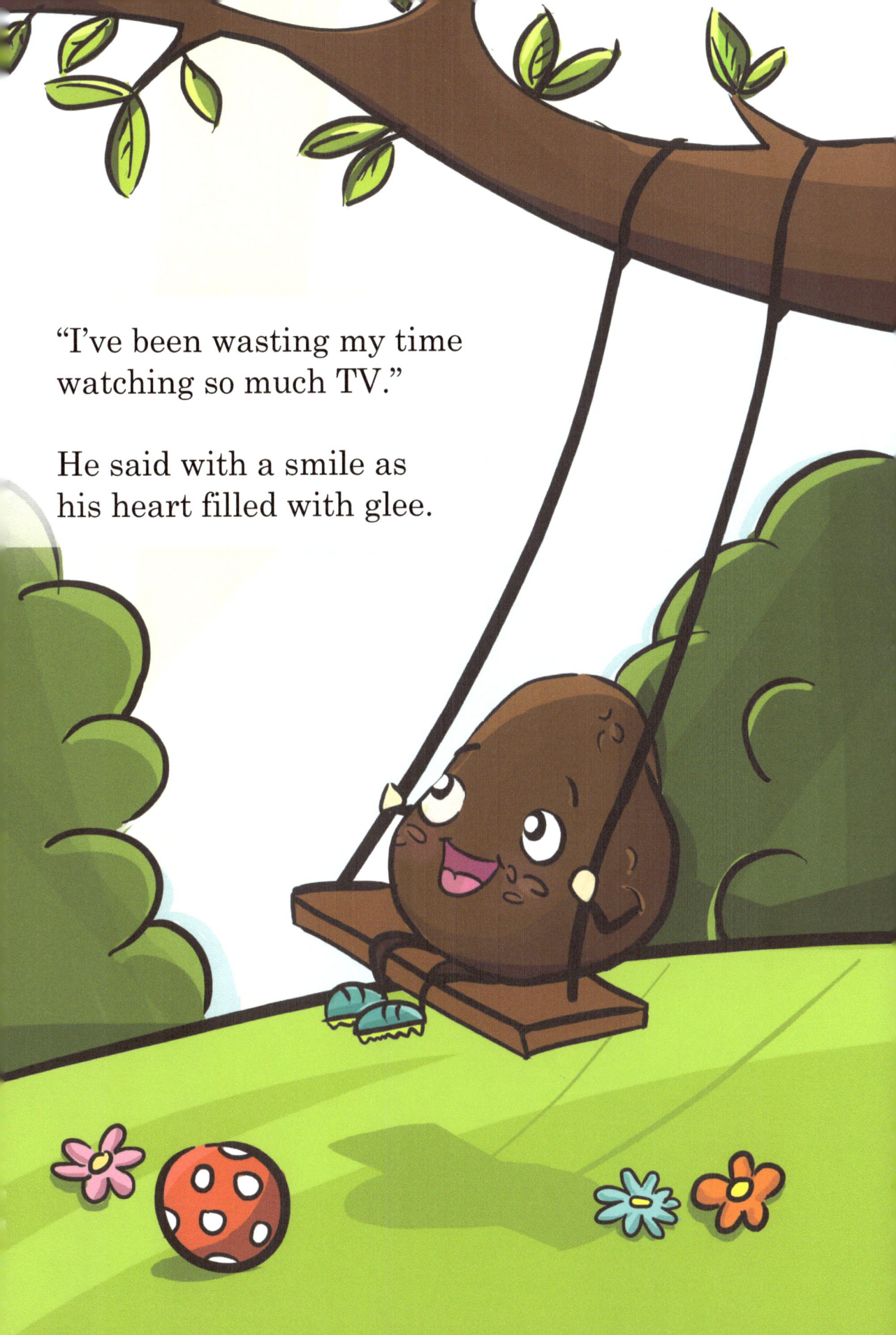

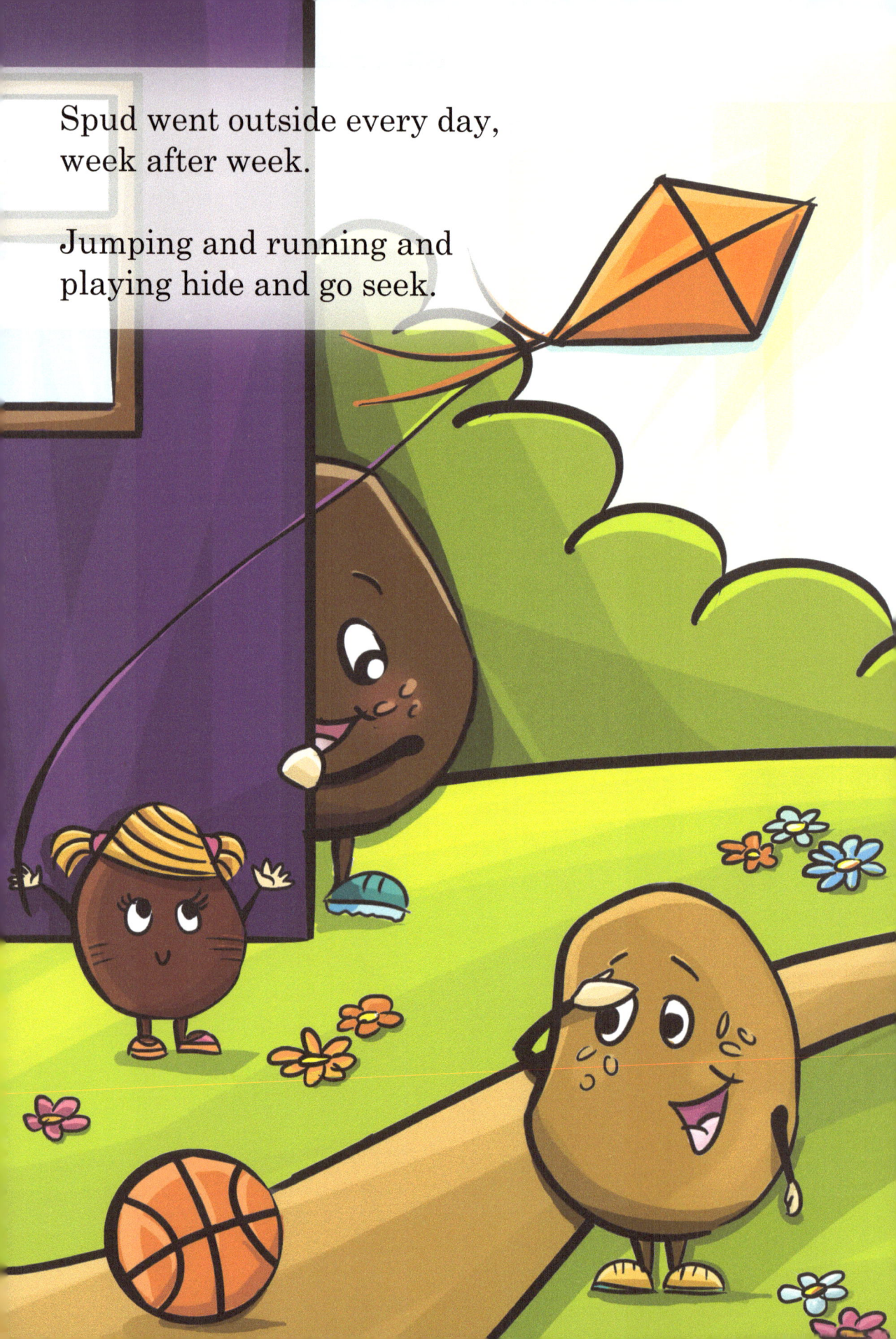

Spud went outside every day,
week after week.

Jumping and running and
playing hide and go seek.

So take it from Spud
the couch loving tater.

It's more fun to be active
and watch TV later.

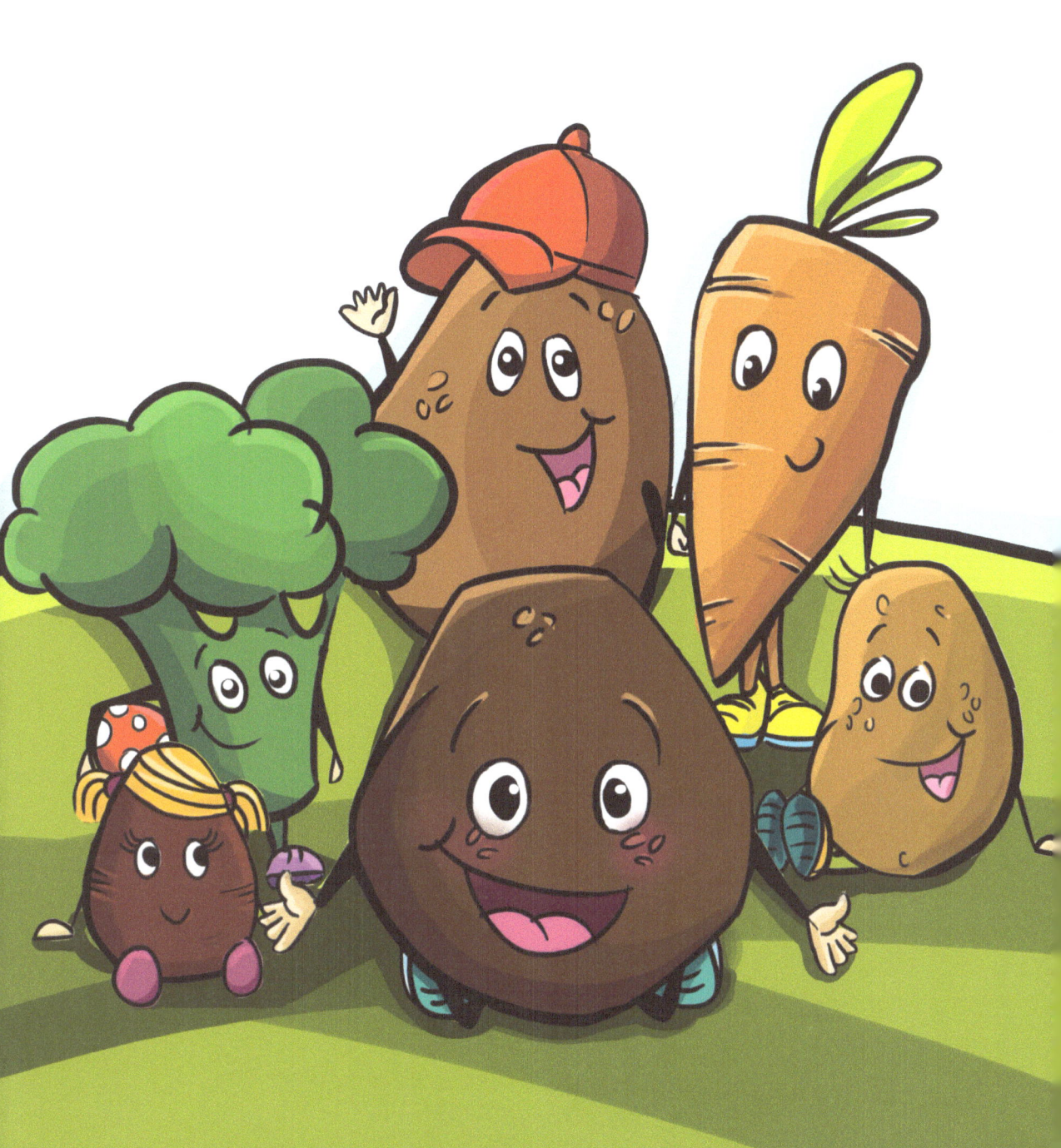

www.ingramcontent.com/pod-product-compliance
Lightning Source LLC
Chambersburg PA
CBHW060818290526
45792CB00005BB/1712